Health Benefits of Oats

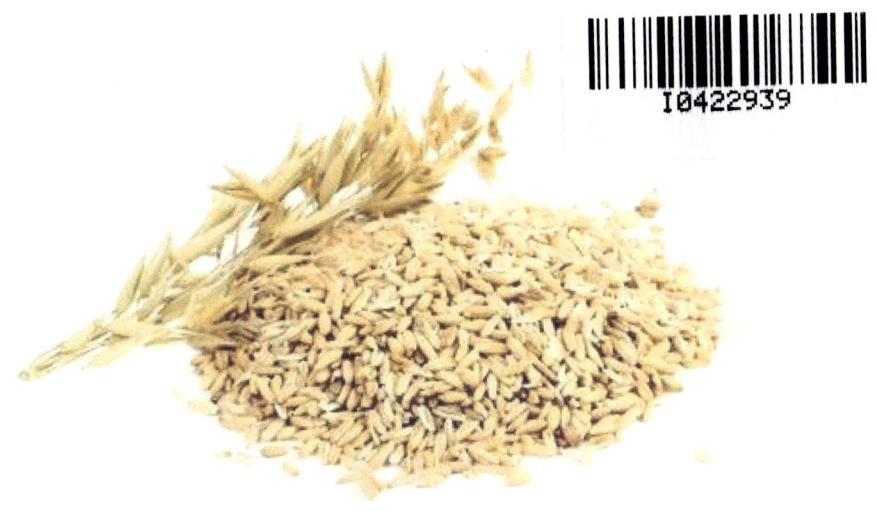

By M. Usman

Health Learning Series

Mendon Cottage Books

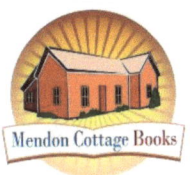

JD-Biz Publishing

Disclaimer

The information is this book is provided for informational purposes only. It is not intended to be used and medical advice or a substitute for proper medical treatment by a qualified health care provider. The information is believed to be accurate as presented based on research by the author.

The contents have not been evaluated by the U.S. Food and Drug Administration or any other Government or Health Organization and the contents in this book are not to be used to treat cure or prevent disease or mental illness.

The author or publisher is not responsible for the use or safety of any diet, procedure or treatment mentioned in this book. The author or publisher is not responsible for errors or omissions that may exist.

Warning

The Book is for informational purposes only and before taking on any diet, treatment or medical procedure it is recommended to consult with your primary care provider.

Our books are available at

1. Amazon.com
2. Barnes and Noble
3. Itunes
4. Kobo
5. Smashwords
6. Google Play Books

Table of Contents

Getting Started

Chapter # 1: Intro

Since the season of scientific researches in the 20th Century, the popularity of oats has been on the rise and they are gaining ever increasing respect in the scientific community as a nutritious diet. Oats are steadily but surely gaining over the breakfast market and each day a great number of people make the switch in search of the perfect breakfast. No doubt, all those cereal commercials hailing oats have a major hand in making people switch to oats too, but if it weren't for its mammoth-like health benefits, oats would never have had a chance to remain in the market.

But before diving straight into the specifics and health benefits of oats it would better to give a basic overview of oats and explain how they became one of the greatest grains on the planet.

The infamous oat, known in the scientific world as *Avena Sativa*, is a grain obtained from a cereal plan, grown for its seeds. The seeds interestingly are also known as oats and are the part of the plant that is mainly consumed; like many other grains, oats grow on stalks with their kernels distributed along a partial tree-like structure. After being harvested, the grains have their tough hulls removed before they can be made available into the market, either as whole or in milled formed.

When it comes to cultivation, oats are one of those plants that are able to withstand poor growing conditions; this is one of the reasons they were cultivated in Europe. Still, the best climate for growing oats is considered to be temperate. Their lower heat requirement during the summers and significant tolerance to wet weather makes them more compatible to variable regions than grains like wheat, barley and rye. On top of this, oats are an annual crop, meaning they can be planted in the autumn for a late summer harvest or during the spring for an early autumn harvest. The resilience & compatibility of oats can be judged by the fact that out of the total world oat produce for 2013, i.e. 21 million tons, Russia and Canada took the top spots with approximately 4 million and 3 million tons of oats respectively.

The modern oats are descendants of the wild ret oat, a plant that originated from within Asia. Oats have been in cultivation in various regions of the world for over 2000 years. Before oats were consumed as a food item, they were being used for their medicinal properties, a use which is now again gaining momentum. The cultivation of oats in Europe is widespread and historically, oat was an important commercial crop for the people of Scotland, Germany, Great Britain and Scandinavian countries.

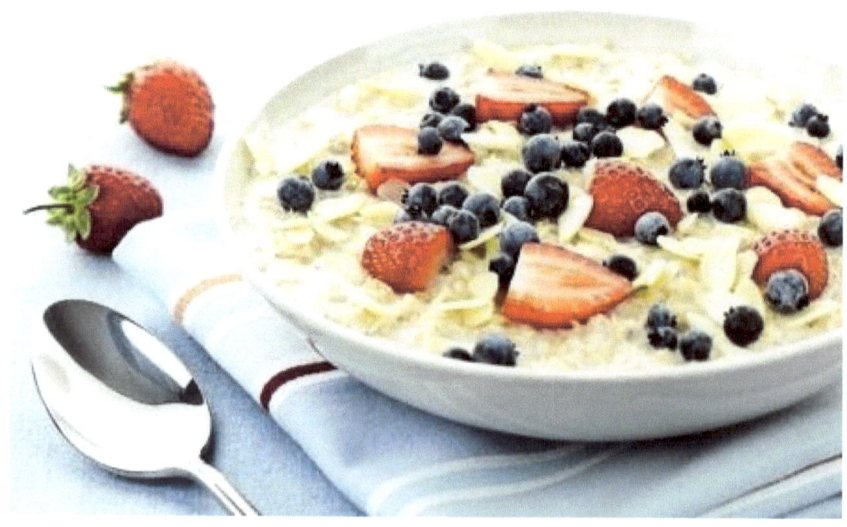

Oats are mainly consumed in the form of porridge, an ingredient in breakfast cereals or in baked goods like oatcakes, oat bread and oat cookies. Since the start of the 21st century, oats have been consumed more because of their nutritious benefits than their taste and as a matter of fact this attitude is not wrong. Here's why:

Oats are a rich source of fiber, calcium, protein, and vitamin E, to name a few minerals. Due to its high fiber content they are an excellent dietary supplement; moreover, the grain can be eaten by all classes due to its variety and inexpensiveness when compared with other grains. Oats contain beta-glucan, which is a type of soluble fiber that prevents very fast absorption of glucose into the blood sugar ensuring lesser blood sugar spikes that otherwise encourage the body to store fats. Oats were and are being used in skin care and cosmetic products; colloidal oat extract has a very soothing effect for the skin. To name a few dermatological products, oat extracts are used in masques, facial cleansers and in skin enhancers. The magnesium mentioned previously is responsible for the normal function of many enzymes used in the process of producing energy in the body. It also aids in preventing heart attacks, strokes, reduces stress on heart muscles and regulates blood pressure.

This is just a glimpse of what's about to come as oat might just be what you're missing.

Chapter # 2: Nutritional Worth

Consumption of oats in the form of oatmeal can provide the body with the essential amount of proteins, calories and fats needed by the body to function properly every day. According to the US department of Agriculture, a single cup of plain oatmeal cooked with water can supply as much as 166 calories, 6 grams of protein and 4 grams of fat. The nutrients found in oats not only provide the sufficient energy to satisfy the body's energy requirement but also help in the maintenance of fluids, muscle mass and cell structure.

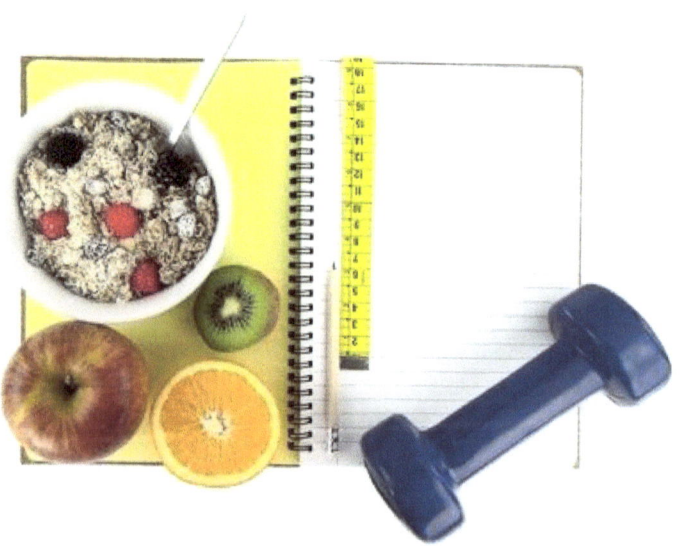

Similar to other grains, oats are also well-known for their dietary content, beta-glucan in their case. Beta-glucan is a type of fiber, unique to oats that can help reduce levels of bad cholesterol in the body. A single cup of oats alone carry 16.5 grams of fiber that is almost half of the body's need per day. Moving over to minerals, oats are packed with the likes of manganese, phosphorous, selenium, fiber, zinc and magnesium. Oats can provide almost half the amount of manganese needed by the body per day; the importance of manganese alone can be judged by the part it plays in the formation of connection tissues, growth of bones, calcium absorption and normal brain function. The other minerals in the list also are vital for the body and are explained in forth coming sections.

A detailed account of the nutritional wellness of oats is given in the following table. The amount per 1 cup taken is 156 grams.

Calorie Information	
Nutrient	**Amount**
Total Calories	607 cal
From Carbohydrates	425 cal
From Fat	90.1 cal
From Proteins	91.2 cal
Carbohydrates	
Nutrient	**Amount**
Total Carbohydrates	103 g
Dietary Fiber	16.5 g
Starch	-
Sugar	-
Fats & Fatty Acids	
Nutrient	**Amount**
Total Fat	10.8 g
Saturated Fat	1.9 g
Mono-saturated Fat	3.4 g
Polyunsaturated Fat	4.0 g

Total Omega-3 Fatty acids	173 mg
Total Omega-6 Fatty acids	3781 mg

Proteins	
Nutrient	**Amount**
Protein	26.4 g

Vitamins	
Nutrient	**Amount**
Vitamin A, C, D, E, K	0 g
Thiamin	1.2 mg
Riboflavin	0.2 mg
Niacin	1.5 mg
Vitamin B6	0.2 mg
Folate	87.4 mcg
Vitamin B12	0.0 mg
Pantothenic Acid	2.1 mg

Minerals	
Nutrient	**Amount**
Calcium	84.3 mg
Iron	7.4 mg
Magnesium	276 mg
Phosphorus	816 mg
Potassium	669 mg
Sodium	3.1 mg
Zinc	6.2 mg
Copper	1.0 mg
Manganese	7.7 mg

Chapter # 3: Types of Oats

Before going into the whole selection & storage criteria, it is better to know the types of oats out in the market, so here are the major types of oats commonly found in the market.

Steel cut oats:

These are oats in their whole form that have been cut into two or three pieces by cutters made of steel so as to make coarse and rough oatmeal. The normal use for steel cut oats is to make oatcakes and traditional porridges.

Jumbo rolled oats/flakes:

These are oats, also in their whole form, that have first been softened with steam and then placed between rollers so flakes can be made out of them. Jumbo rolled oats find their use in muesli or in thick porridges.

Rolled oats:

Rolled oats are a variant of steel cut oats that are first softened using steam and then rolled to produce flakes. They are smaller in size than jumbo flakes and so are quicker to cool, thus making a smoother, finer porridge. They are generally found in sachets in supermarkets. A mix of jumbo and rolled oats is used to make oatcakes, biscuits and cereal bars.

Oatmeal:

Oatmeal is one of the most popular variant of oats; it is made by using grooved rolls to break up the oats so they can be classified, from coarse oatmeal to fine oatmeal. Before the invention of rolled oats, porridge was made from oatmeal. Oatmeal porridge takes longer to cook but is much thicker in texture in comparison with rolled oats. Oatmeal finds use in oatcakes, biscuits, cones and various toppings.

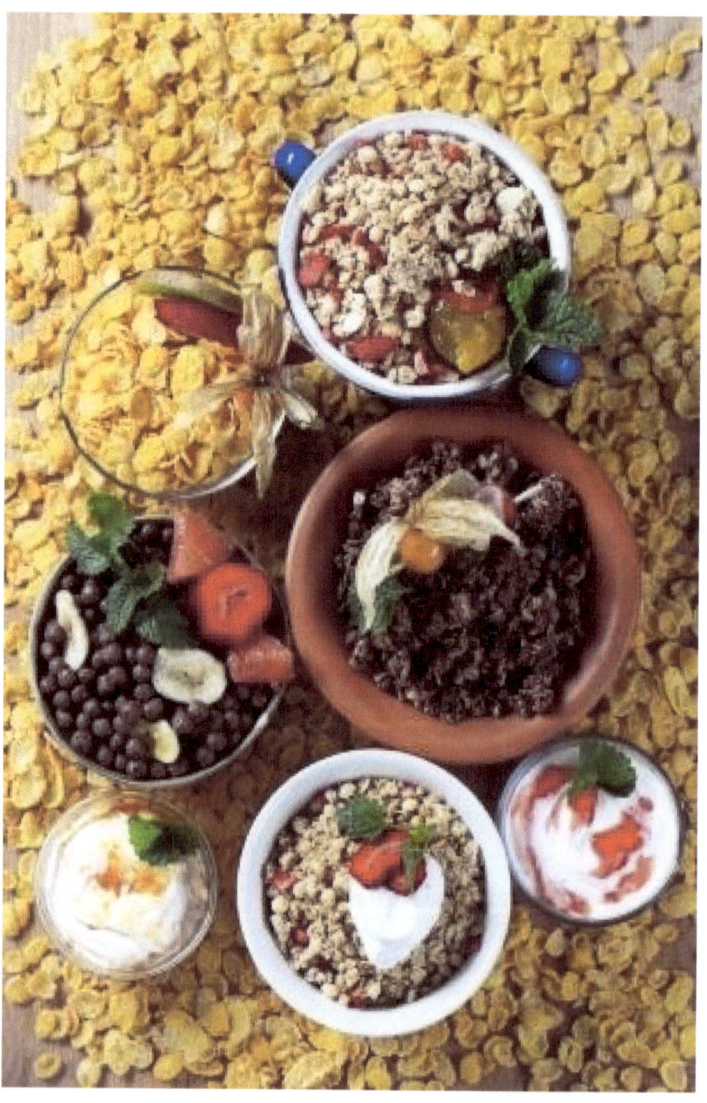

Oat flour:

Oat flour is much finer than oatmeal and is made by finely grinding and sieving the oats. The texture of the flour can vary from rough to smooth depending on the grinding quality. Oat flour is commonly used in making cakes and breads.

Oat Bran:

This is not exactly oat but rather the outer casing of the oat grain that is very high in fiber. It can be purchased from local health stores.

Chapter # 4: Selection & Storage

Oats are available in both bulk and in pre-packaged forms. When buying in bulk, make sure that just as with any other grain, the container is covered and is free of any debris; also choose a store with a high turnover rate as this will ensure maximum freshness. After choosing a good store for purchasing oats in bulk, smell the oats to make sure they are fresh. One thing you should be certain of is that there should be no moisture in or around the container whether you are purchasing bulk or pre-packaged oats. Also when compared to other grains, oats have a slightly higher fat content making them more probable to going rancid.

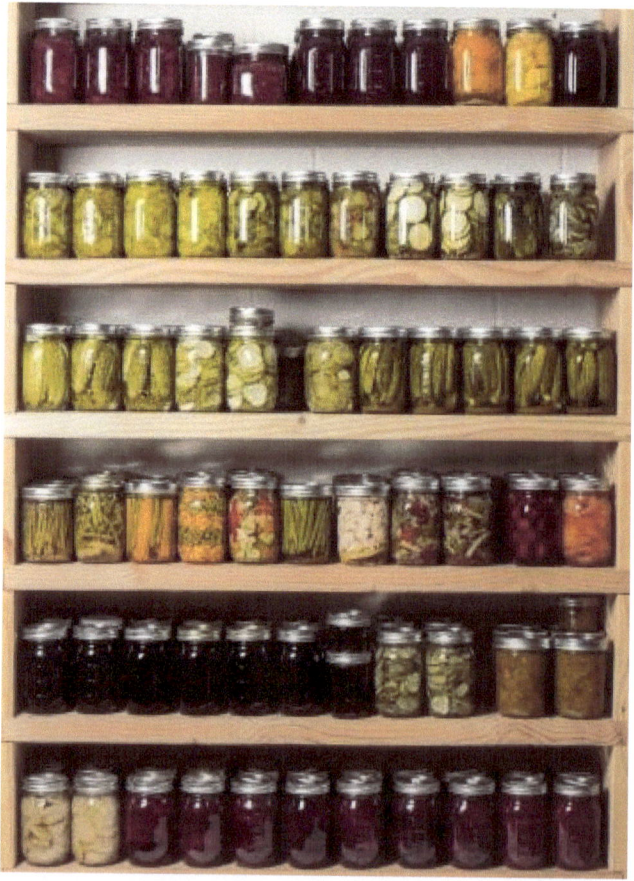

When it comes to storing, oats should be kept in an airtight container that should be set aside in a cool, dark and dry place. It should also be noticed that the place where oats are stored should have minimum chance of vermin intrusion and minimum changes in temperature as temperature changes tend to condensate the moisture in the container allowing molds to develop much more rapidly. The oats may be stored for a period of 3 months and can be further refrigerated to 6 months.

How to tell if Oatmeal has gone bad or rotten?

Although not completely accurate, the body's senses are still very reliable instruments for judging the staleness of oats. Dry oats in the form of oatmeal can last for several years so before you blindly consume oats, its best to make sure that they have not gone bad. If the oats start to reek with any odor or taste different than usual, spit the oats right out and discard them. Prepared oatmeal can be distinguished when it goes bad by looking at the level of separateness of the liquid in a serving of oatmeal.

Chapter # 5: Are Oats Gluten-Free?

Before moving onto the recipes, this very important question that concerns a huge percentage of the population remains unanswered. Are Oats Gluten Free?

Gluten, in the simplest words is a mixture of two types of proteins that are present in cereal grains; this mixture is responsible for giving the characteristic feature of elasticity to dough made of that cereal. Gluten is commonly found in wheat, rye and barley and it is unknowingly one of the most loved compounds as it is what gives are favorite foods that special touch we most cherish; it makes pizza stretchy, bread spongy and thickens sauces & soups.

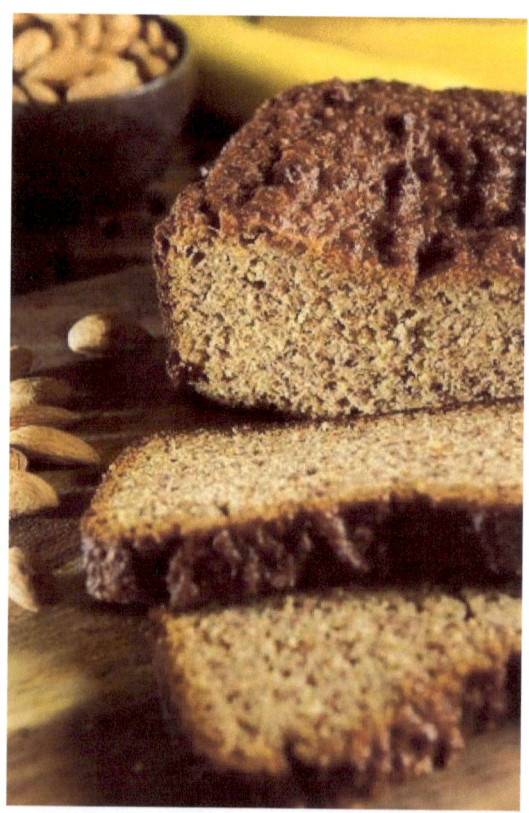

Some people are gluten-intolerant that can be defined as a condition when the body produces an abnormal response on the breakdown of gluten in the intestines. The most commonly known form of gluten-intolerance is the celiac disease; when a person with celiac disease consumes gluten, the immune system of the person's body sends out a signal that triggers a hormonal response damaging the intestines; the damage done by the hormones further results in the failure to absorb vital nutrients from the food consumed. According to the US National Institute of Health, celiac disease almost affects one in every 141 people and the numbers are only increasing. In cases of gluten intolerance, doctors recommend a gluten-free diet, meaning patients are unable to consume food items such as wheat, rye, millet and bear, etc. Sometimes the list also includes oats which has lead many gluten-intolerant people to avoid eating oat or oat products. The short answer to the question is No; oats do not contain gluten and are in most cases safe for people with gluten intolerance.

The main problem with oats and their alleged gluten content is contamination. Oats on their own do not contain any gluten, as in wheat or other grains but when oats are processed commercially they are often treated in facilities that deal with grains like wheat as well. The gluten in these grains contaminates oats and the nature of gluten intolerance is such that even the smallest trace of gluten can cause severe discomfort. Secondly, contamination can also happen on the field where oats are grown alongside wheat. Contamination can vary greatly between different batches of processed oats therefore, one box may be okay but the other of the same brand may not be.

Still gluten free oats are available commercially and they are among the least expensive gluten free grains in the market too. Thus, it is preferred that if you are gluten intolerant, it is best to buy gluten free oats and not take any chances. The following is a list of oat meals that are gluten free and can be used as an alternate if you are gluten-intolerant:

Bob's Red Mill:

> This brand produces three types of gluten free oatmeal that include quick-cooking oats, steel cut oats and rolled oats. The company tests the oat for gluten down to 20 parts per million making the possibility of consuming gluten very little.

GF Harvests:

> GF Harvests is a business owned by a family who themselves suffer from celiac disease. Oats are grown by the company and undergo extensive tests to make sure that oats are uncontaminated. They even test the seeds to 3 parts per million; GF harvests holds gluten free certification and produce organic gluten-free oats and regular gluten free oats.

Holly's Oatmeal:

> Holly's oatmeal also produces one of the purest possible oatmeal with testing for gluten being up to 5 parts per million. Along with producing gluten-free oatmeal, Holly's also produces two flavors of the oatmeal; plain and cranberry. The oatmeal is available online in addition to the market.

Health Benefits of Oats

Chapter # 6: Lowers Cholesterol Levels

Cholesterol problems are some of the greatest ailments swiftly taking over the modern population. The fast-paced, head-on competitive life has often left people forgotten about their health and sinking into the array of diseases originating from high levels of cholesterol.

A high level of cholesterol are acutely responsible for the build-up of plaques in the blood vessels; if these plaques by even the slightest chance get damaged or grow too much of size, they can break and block the whole of the blood vessel, effectively cutting off the flow of blood, causing blood clots, stroke or in a worst-case scenario, a heart attack. This explains the need for lowering cholesterol levels in order to reduce the risk of cardiovascular diseases.

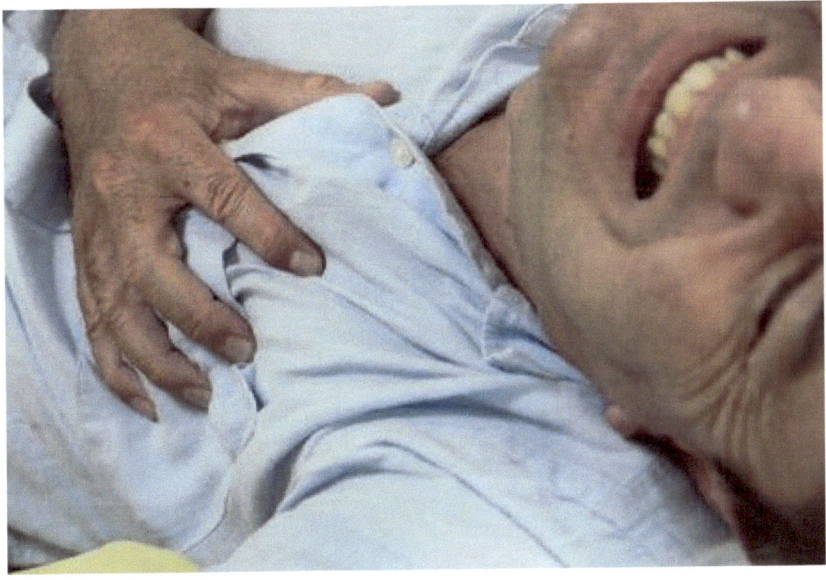

A hot, steaming bowl of oatmeal can help you achieve the objective of lowering cholesterol, along with being the perfect way to kick off your day. Oats, oatmeal or oat bran, all contain a particular type of fiber called beta-glucan. The name might not interest you but it has been of much curiosity for medical researchers. Since 1963, a string of studies have revealed the beneficial effects of beta-glucan; one such study showed that when individuals having cholesterol levels above 220 mg/dl were given soluble oat supplements weighing just 3 grams, on a daily basis, the cholesterol levels were lowered by 8-23%. It should further be noted that a 1% drop in cholesterol accounts for a 2% decrease in the risk of developing heart disease.

Another study that was published in Archives of Internal Medicine confirmed the cholesterol lowering effects of oats when 10,000 American adults were subjected to a study that was tracked for 19 years. After the specified time period, results showed that the people who consumed the most amount of fiber, i.e. 21 grams a day had 12% less coronary heart disease & 11% less cardiovascular diseases. The results were even better with those who ate water-soluble dietary fiber, with a 15% and 10% reduction in coronary heart disease and cardiovascular diseases respectively.

Chapter # 7: Enhances Overall Cardiovascular Health

Oats, which are already known for removing cholesterol through the body through their high fiber content, are now being found to have a second protective mechanism for cardiovascular health. Antioxidants called avenanthramides, unique to the likes of oats help prevent heart diseases by eliminating free radicals that damage good cholesterol in the body. A study conducted at Tufts University, published in The Journal of Nutrition showed the antioxidant effects of avenanthramides in protecting LDL cholesterol by carrying experiments on lab animals with similar bodily function to that of humans. After a 0.25 grams dose of oat-bran, it took only 40 minutes for avenanthramides to appear in blood tests showing that avenanthramides had successfully made its way into the blood stream. Next, the researchers tested to see the effectiveness of avenanthramides in preventing the oxidation of good cholesterol by free radicals of copper. Not only did avenanthramides increase the time before cholesterol got oxidized but when supplements of vitamin C were added the duration was extended to 216 minutes from 137 minutes. This was a major breakthrough that gave the green signal to many other studies on the cardiovascular benefits of oats.

A study published in the Journal of Family Practice showed that oats were particularly handy when it came to controlling the blood pressure. Using a randomized, controlled methodology, researchers subjected 18 hyperinsulemic and hypertensive men & women for six weeks. Half of the group was given oat cereal while the other half were given a cereal with a lower fiber percentage. The group with the oat cereal enjoyed a 7.5 mmHg decrease in maximum blood pressure and a 5.5 mmHg decrease in minimum blood pressure.

Another chemical that is very useful for the body and is found in oats is lignan. As lignans make their way into the intestines they are converted into mammalian lignans; one of these mammalian lignans is called enterolactone, which is a chemical known to protect against hormone dependent ailments like cancers and heart disease. A Danish study focused on the concentration of enterolactone by analyzing the blood samples of 800 women and found out those women who consumed the most amounts of oats on a daily basis had a higher concentration of enterolactone in their blood; the study was published in Journal of Nutrition.

Benefits for Postmenopausal women:

Whole grains such as oats are very vital for the cardiovascular health of postmenopausal women who have high cholesterol levels, blood pressure or other cardiovascular problems. A study that was published in the 2014 issue of Nutrition Journal revealed that oatmeal increased the antioxidant protection level in older postmenopausal women. It also halted a chronic inflammation that had been linked to the development of cancer and heart diseases. The researchers specifically aimed this study at post-menopausal women as they wished to study the association between inflammation and aging, and further because age-related lack of estrogen had been found to contribute to oxidative stress. The team found out that oatmeal extracts not only had well-pronounced anti-inflammatory effects but also was free of any side effects. This result was especially ground-breaking as other non-steroidal anti-inflammatory drugs also reduced inflammation but at the same time interfered with the body's own healing process.

Chapter # 8: Lowers Type-II Diabetes Risk

Oat being a whole grain is a rich source of the mineral magnesium; as it was stated in the previous section, magnesium is a mineral which acts as a helping compound for more than 300 enzymes involved in reactions in different parts of the body.

The United States FDA permits only food items that contain at least 51% whole grain content by weight to display a health claim regarding heart disease and cancers. Research suggests that consumption of whole grains like oats on a daily basis can reduce the risk of type 2 diabetes. The research was published in the 2008 issue of Diabetes care whose purpose was to find the relation between intakes of magnesium with the risk of type 2 diabetes in African-American women. The trial lasted for 8 years and was carried out on 41,186 participants; the risk of type 2 diabetes was found to be 31% lower in women who frequently ate oats, in one form or another, compared to those who didn't consume any or minimal amount of any whole food item. But when the experiment was carried out with magnesium supplements the rate of reduction dropped down to 19%, indicating that there was indeed the combination of minerals and compounds in whole grains that kept the rate even lower.

A research was carried out by scientists in Mannheim, Germany on dietary intervention on 14 people with uncontrolled diabetes and insulin resistance. During a short hospital stay, each patient was introduced to a diabetes optimized diet consisting of oatmeal. Each patient was examined after 4 weeks and it was established that patients were able to achieve a 40% reduction in insulin dosage which lasted even after the trial ended, without any interference from doctors.

As it was previously stated that magnesium is not the only thing at work in reducing the risk of diabetes, it must also be known that beta-glucan, the fiber present in oats has also been found to have a positive effect on insulin sensitivity. A study published in European Journal of Clinical Nutrition targeted 97 men & women to check for insulin sensitivity. Half the group was given beta-glucan supplements in the form of oats while the other half was kept on control foods. At the end of the trial the control group had no change whatsoever in their sensitivity levels whereas the oat group was found to have an improvement in insulin sensitivity.

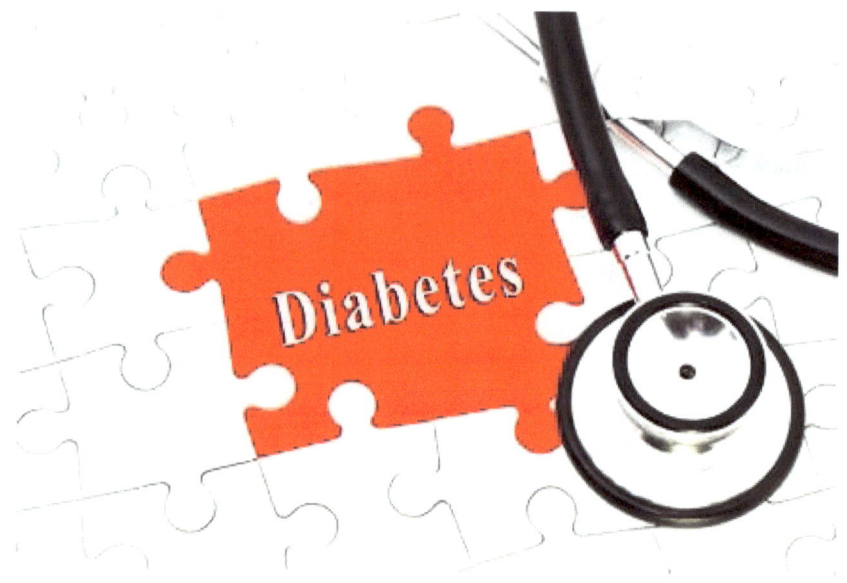

Chapter # 9: Inhibits Cancer

Cancer is swiftly becoming one of the most feared diseases on the planet; it is characterized by out-of-control multiplication of cells and can originate in any part of the body. Cancers harm the body by forming lumps or pile of unhealthy tissues called tumors that grow and interfere with the normal functions of the body. But the real danger begins when a cancerous cell manages to travel to different organs of the body and destroy healthy tissues; over there it replicates itself and feeds on every healthy tissue that once thrived in the body.

Even though, scientists have found many ways to halt the spread of these cells and in many cases destroy them, they still haven't found a permanent, effective solution that would put an end to the risk of cancer. Moreover, the solutions found have too many side-effects, therefore they can only be used when it is sure that a person has cancer and not to reduce its risk in the first place.

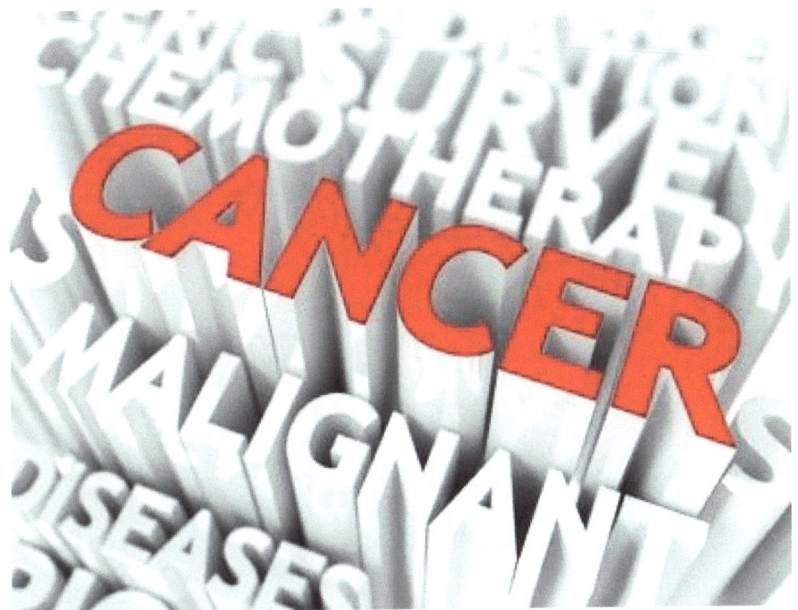

Researchers have found fiber to be a solid weapon against cancer and time and again whole grains like oats that are filled with fiber have proved this point. A study published in the International Journal of Epidemiology, aimed at studying the effects of whole grains in limiting breast cancer targeted about 36,000 pre-menopausal women. It was found that out of the many nutrients present in whole grains, fiber was the most effective one. Women who ate at least 13g of fiber a day reduced their risk of breast cancer by 41 percent compared to those who ate only 4 grams a day; an increased intake of fiber, i.e. 30 grams/day brought the risk further down to 48%. In addition, it was found that pre-menopausal women, whose diet consisted of at least 6g of fiber from fruit sources, had a reduced risk of breast cancer by 29%. This concluded that 13 grams of fiber from grains such as oats and 6 grams of fiber from fruits provided the optimum combo for bringing down the risk of cancer.

The fiber content of oats has been given in the previous section; the fiber content of fruits is as follows:

Food	Fiber Content in Grams
Apple	5.0
Banana	4.0
Blueberries	3.92
Orange	4.42
Pear	5.02
Prunes	3.02

Strawberries	3.82
Raspberries	8.36

When it comes to postmenopausal women, a study showed that women who consumed the most cereal (oatmeal) had a 50% reduction in the risk of developing breast cancer. The prospective study was carried out on 51,000 postmenopausal women for about 8 years and showed a 34% reduction in breast cancer risk for those women consuming only fiber from fruit, while a 50% reduction in those eating oats. The study was published in the 2008, January issue of the International Journal of Cancer.

Breast cancer was not the only cancer that was suppressed by the addition of oats in ones diet; colorectal cancer was also slowed down by following a diet rich in fiber, especially the one found in oats. For those who are unaware of colorectal cancer; it is a cancer that forms in both the colon and the rectum; it is often referred to as bowel cancer and is the most commonly occurring type of cancer, according to the UK National Health Service.

Researchers in Britain and the Netherlands pooled all available research on the link between colorectal cancer and fiber consumption. The findings were published in November issue of BMJ. The link between reduced risk of cardiovascular disease and fiber consumption had already been developed but it was the one between colorectal cancer and fiber that needed to be established. To find out such a link, the researchers analyzed the results of 25 studies that had a total of 2 million participants; to remove any inclination towards a study, the design and quality of the study was considered. The researchers ranked the participants in accordance with the amount of fiber they consumed daily and found out that each 10g/day increase in total dietary fiber resulted in a 10% decrease in the risk of colorectal cancer. Another analysis revealed that addition of 3 servings (90g) of oatmeal to the diet resulted in a 20% decrease in the risk. They also confirmed that fiber from fruits and vegetables was not equivalent to that from whole grains as studies showed an inconsistent decrease in the rate of reducing cancer risk when fiber from fruit was consumed instead of grains.

Chapter # 10: Combats Childhood Asthma

Asthma is an incurable disease that affects the normal function of airways in the lungs; the walls of these airways get swollen making the airways highly sensitive to any activity within these walls resulting in a swift allergic reaction to even the smallest irritation. Inflammation results in narrowing of the airways, causing hissing sounds while breathing, chest tightness and other breathing difficulties. Childhood asthma is just like asthma in adults but unlike adults, children don't handle an asthma attack well which often results in trips to the emergency wards and subsequently absentees from school. Even though asthma is incurable, if it is countered from the start, it would be much more comfortable for the child in his/her older days.

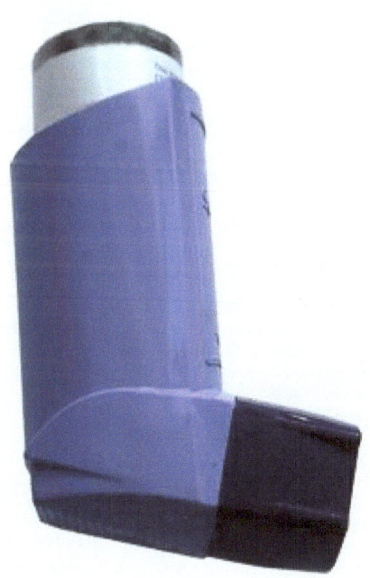

According to the American Lung Association, a whopping 20 million American citizen suffer from asthma; this number is responsible for about 14 million absentees a year from school that adds up to an economic cost of about 16 Billion Dollars an year. An international study on Allergy and Asthma in children suggested that an increased consumption of whole grains like oats and foods like fish could reduce the risk of asthma in children by 50%. The team was from the Dutch National Institute of Public Health and from the Environment Utrecht University Groningen. The team distributed questionnaires to parents with children between the ages of 8-13. Again no association was found between asthma and intake of fruits & vegetables but with children who consumed a high amount of whole grains such as oats had only 4.2% prevalence in wheezing compared to those who consumed little quantities.

Another study was carried out on infants to study the relation between early introductions of complementary foods and the development of allergies like asthma by the age of 5 years. A total of 3781 consecutively born children were made a part of this research and the dietary exposures were studied with respect to time. Allergies like eczema, asthma and rhinitis were assessed using questionnaires while antibodies were analyzed using serum samples when the child reached the age of 5. It was found that introduction of whole grains like rye, wheat and oats at 5 months decreased the risk of asthma and rhinitis while introduction of these foods before the 4th month resulted in an increased risk of eczema. Conclusively, it was found that early introduction of whole foods especially oats decreased the child's risk of developing allergies like asthma.

Conclusion

Once known as fodder for farm animals and food for the poor class is now hastily being accepted at every level in the society. Knowingly or unknowingly, for centuries the lower class has been reaping all the benefits of oats and kept most diseases at bay even without any fancy treatments. Everything to know about oats has been disclosed in this book and now that you've completed it, it can surely be hoped that you'll use the knowledge acquired to incorporate the mega nutritious package into your diet and reap all of its short-term as well as long lasting benefits, to lead a healthy, satisfying life.

Stay safe!

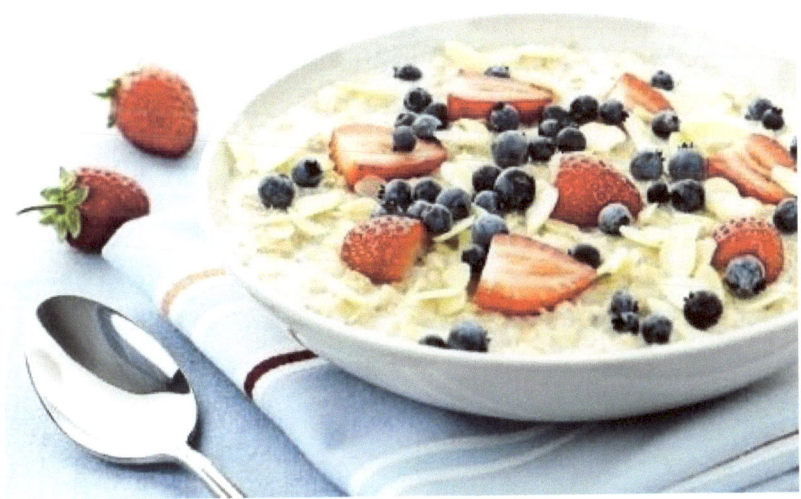

References

1. http://www.123rf.com/photo_16015633_whole-oats-with-ears-isolated-on-white-background.html
2. http://www.123rf.com/photo_7776449_bowl-of-hot-oatmeal-breakfast-cereal-with-fresh-berries.html
3. http://www.123rf.com/photo_11801631_healthy-eating-book.html
4. http://www.123rf.com/photo_24138792_various-types-of-breakfast-cereal--overhead.html
5. http://www.123rf.com/photo_15014637_shelves-of-homemade-preserves-and-canned-goods.html
6. http://www.123rf.com/photo_2669487_gluten-free-banana-almond-bread.html
7. http://www.fotolia.com/id/7456661
8. http://www.fotolia.com/id/35435335
9. http://www.fotolia.com/id/39611032
10. http://www.fotolia.com/id/47533987
11. http://www.fotolia.com/id/49549245

Author Bio

Muhammad Usman is a distinguished medical graduate of Allama iqbal medical college (AIMC). He is a professional writer who has been in the field for more than 4 years. During this time he has produced 10,000+ articles, blogs and eBooks on various niches related to diseases, health, fitness, nutrition and well-being. He is a regular contributor to several journals related to medicine and surgery. He is the editor of several journals and newspapers.

Check out some of the other Health Learning Series books at Amazon.com

Health Learning Series on Amazon

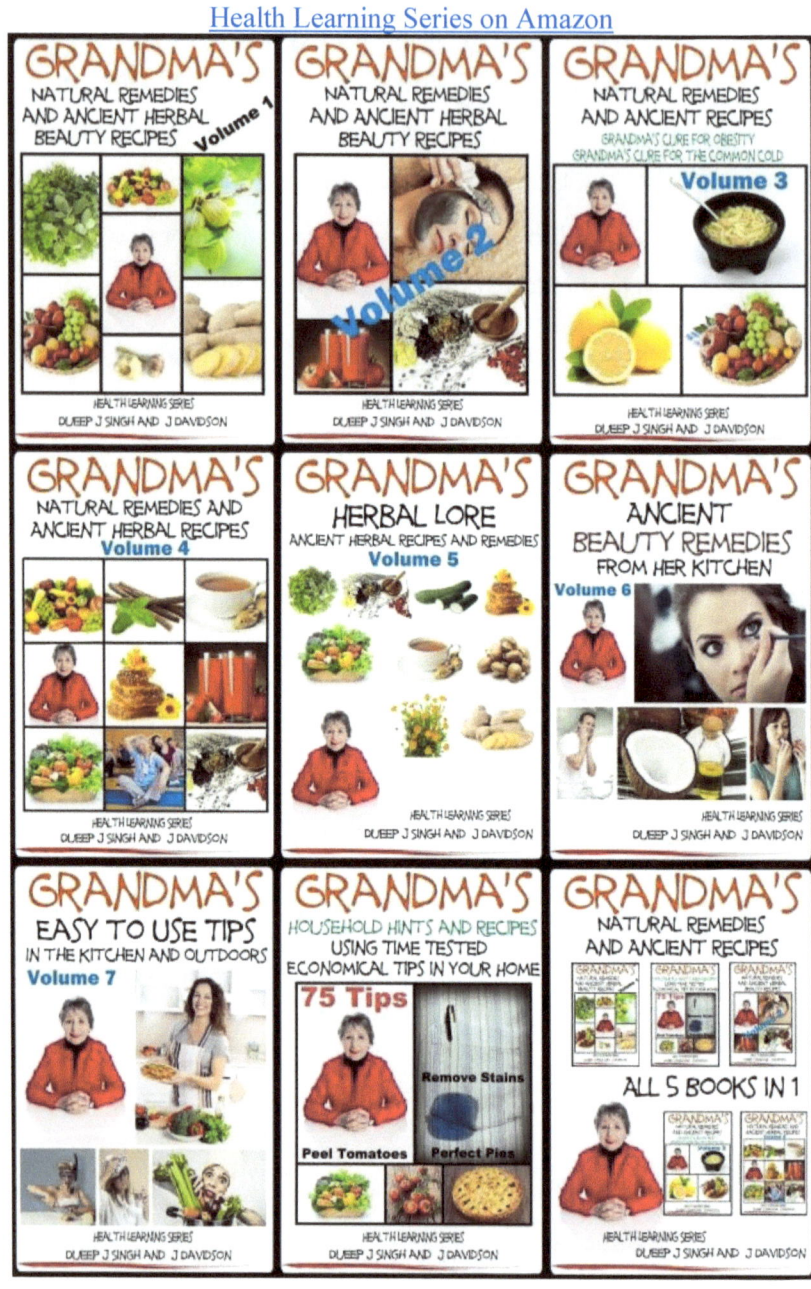

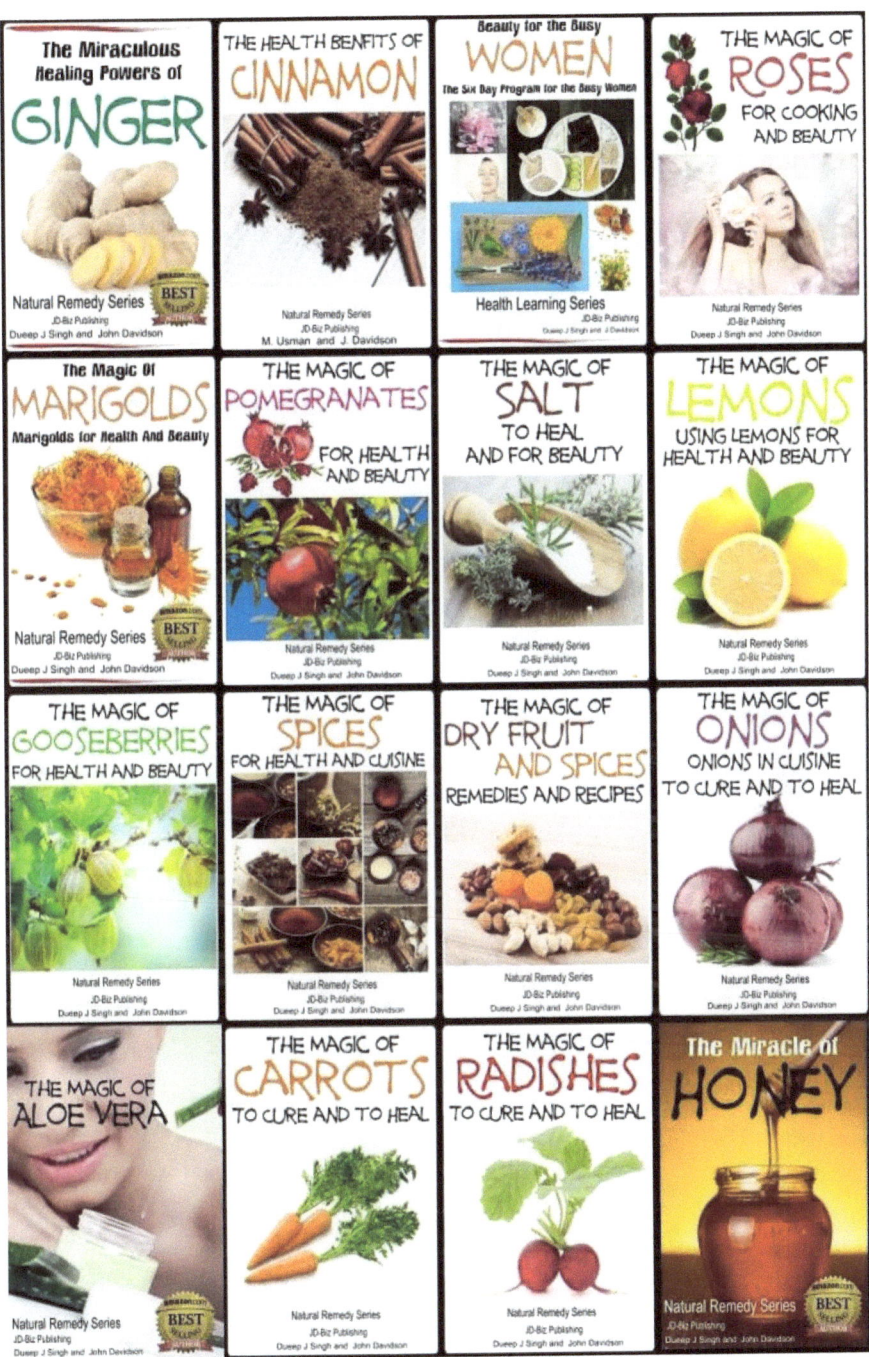

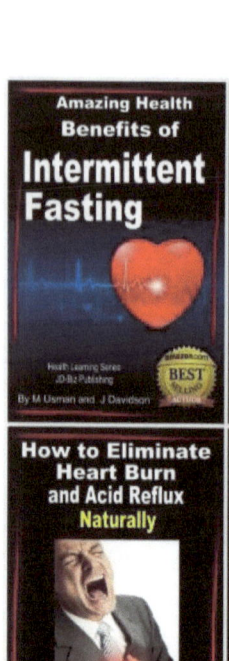

Amazing Health
Benefits of
Intermittent Fasting

Health Learning Series
JD-Biz Publishing
By M Usman and J Davidson

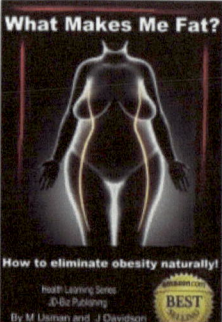

What Makes Me Fat?

How to eliminate obesity naturally!

Health Learning Series
JD-Biz Publishing
By M Usman and J Davidson

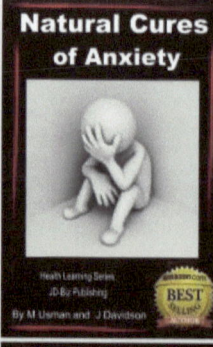

Natural Cures of Anxiety

Health Learning Series
JD-Biz Publishing
By M Usman and J Davidson

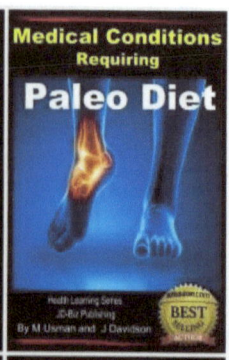

Medical Conditions Requiring
Paleo Diet

Health Learning Series
JD-Biz Publishing
By M Usman and J Davidson

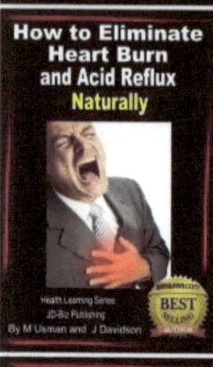

How to Eliminate Heart Burn and Acid Reflux Naturally

Health Learning Series
JD-Biz Publishing
By M Usman and J Davidson

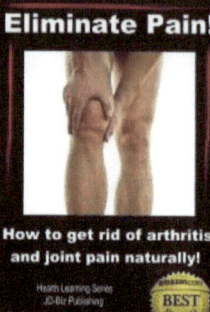

Eliminate Pain!

How to get rid of arthritis and joint pain naturally!

Health Learning Series
JD-Biz Publishing
By M Usman and J Davidson

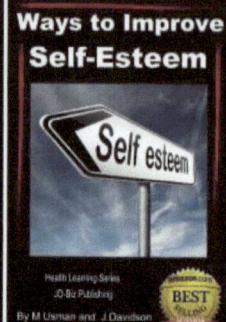

Ways to Improve Self-Esteem

Health Learning Series
JD-Biz Publishing
By M Usman and J Davidson

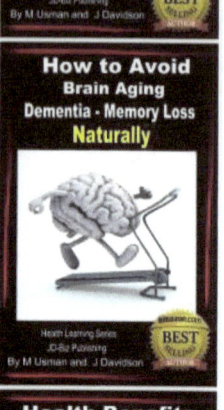

How to Avoid Brain Aging
Dementia - Memory Loss
Naturally

Health Learning Series
JD-Biz Publishing
By M Usman and J Davidson

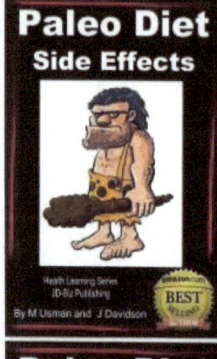

Paleo Diet Side Effects

Health Learning Series
JD-Biz Publishing
By M Usman and J Davidson

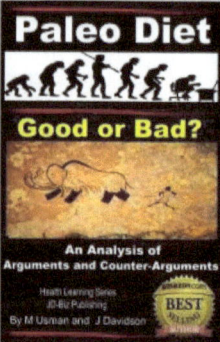

Paleo Diet

Good or Bad?

An Analysis of Arguments and Counter-Arguments

Health Learning Series
JD-Biz Publishing
By M Usman and J Davidson

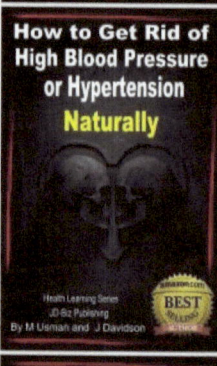

How to Get Rid of High Blood Pressure or Hypertension Naturally

Health Learning Series
JD-Biz Publishing
By M Usman and J Davidson

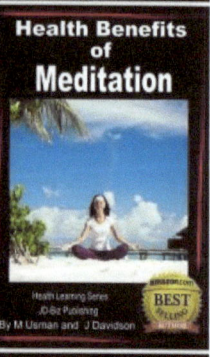

Health Benefits of Meditation

Health Learning Series
JD-Biz Publishing
By M Usman and J Davidson

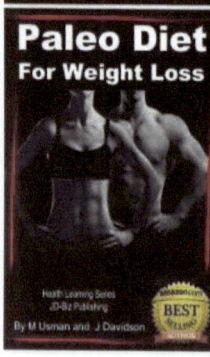

Paleo Diet For Weight Loss

Health Learning Series
JD-Biz Publishing
By M Usman and J Davidson

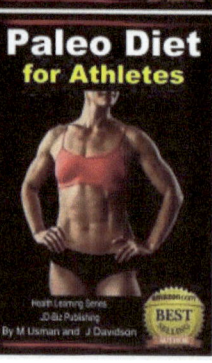

Paleo Diet for Athletes

Health Learning Series
JD-Biz Publishing
By M Usman and J Davidson

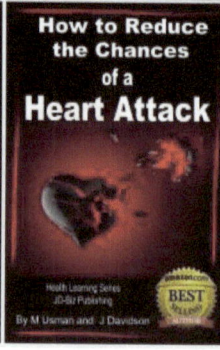

How to Reduce the Chances of a Heart Attack

Health Learning Series
JD-Biz Publishing
By M Usman and J Davidson

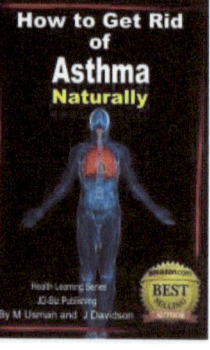

How to Get Rid of Asthma Naturally

Health Learning Series
JD-Biz Publishing
By M Usman and J Davidson

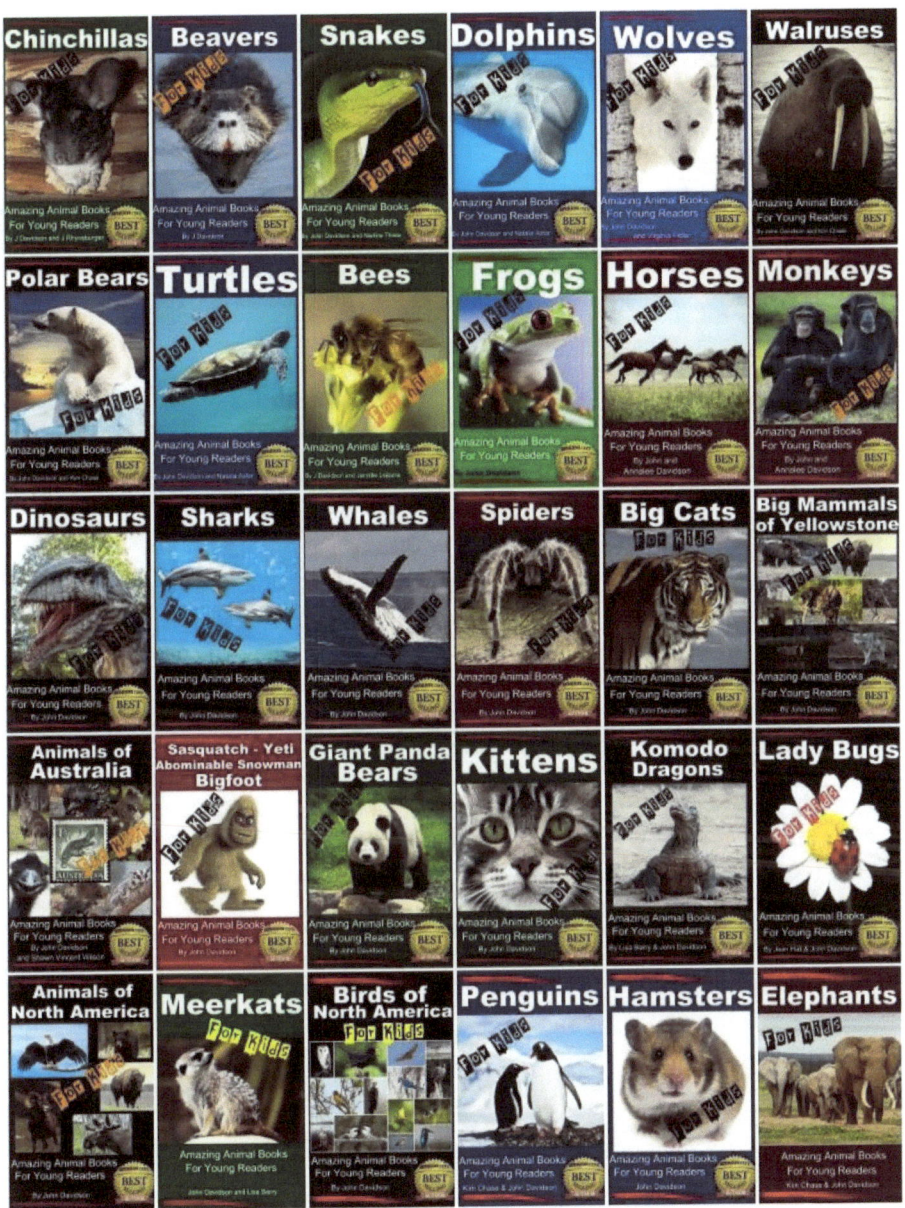

Learn To Draw Series

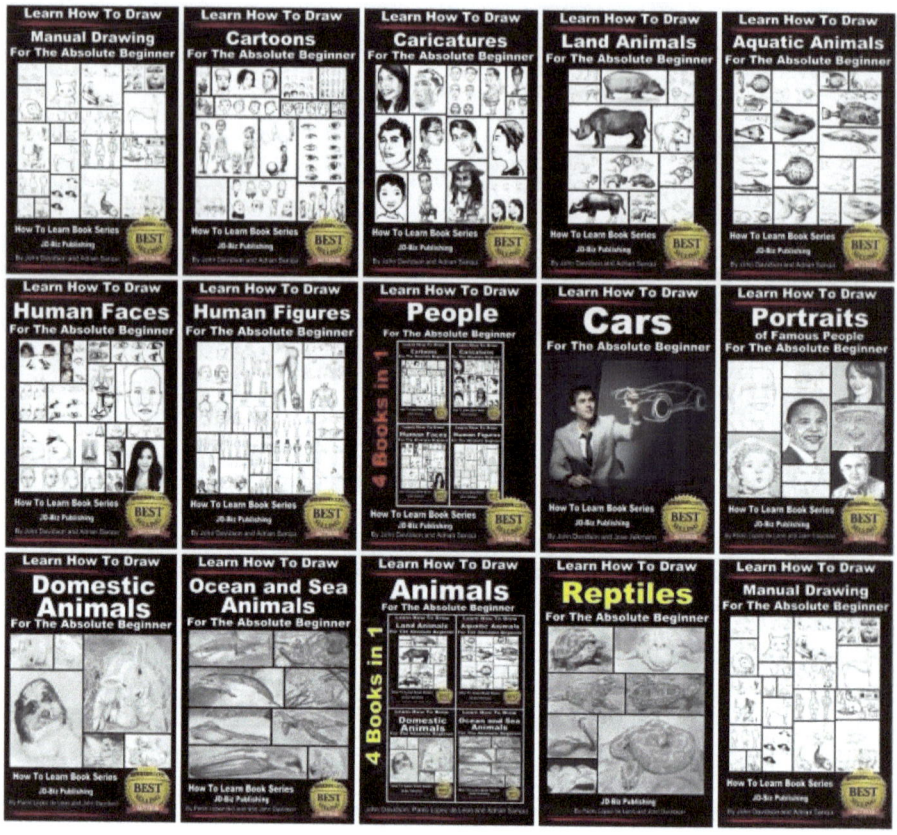

How to Build and Plan Books

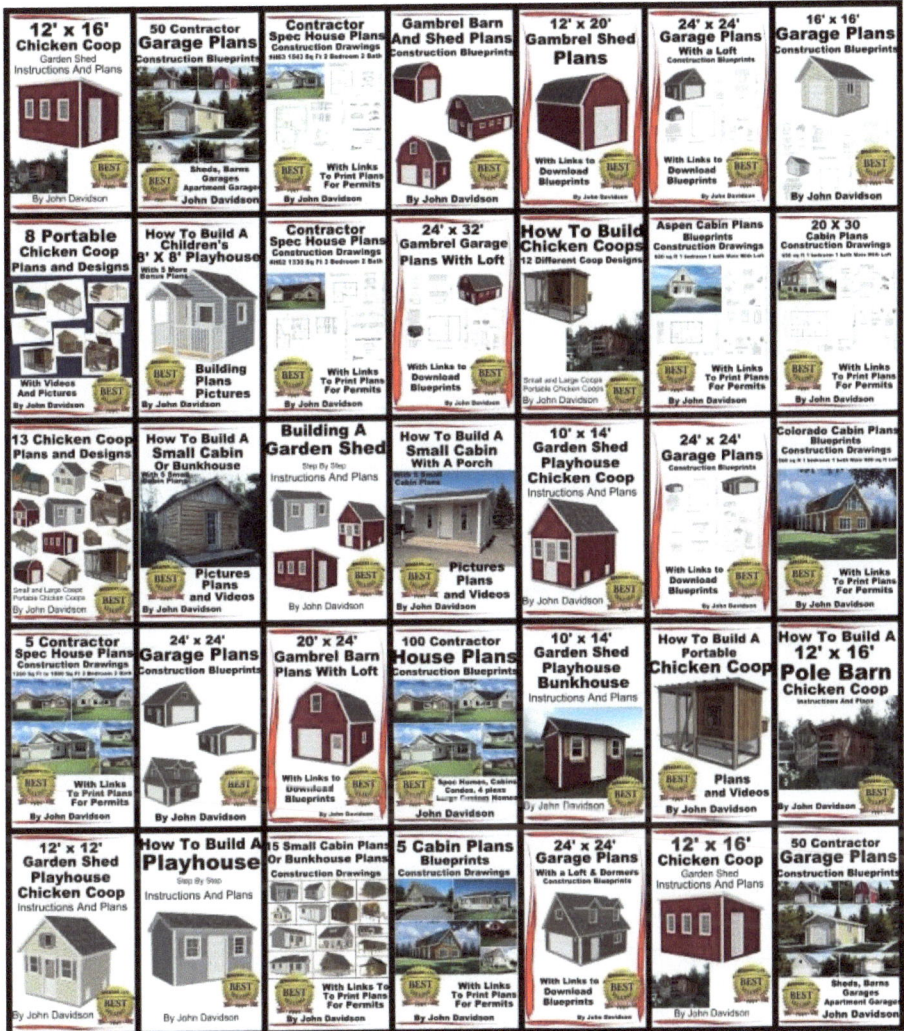

Our books are available at

1. Amazon.com
2. Barnes and Noble
3. Itunes
4. Kobo
5. Smashwords
6. Google Play Books

Download Free Books!

http://MendonCottageBooks.com

Publisher

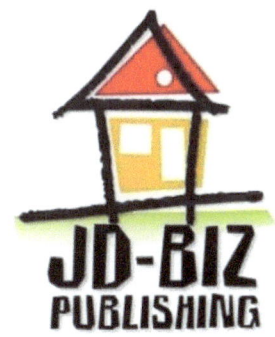

JD-Biz Corp

P O Box 374

Mendon, Utah 84325

http://www.jd-biz.com/

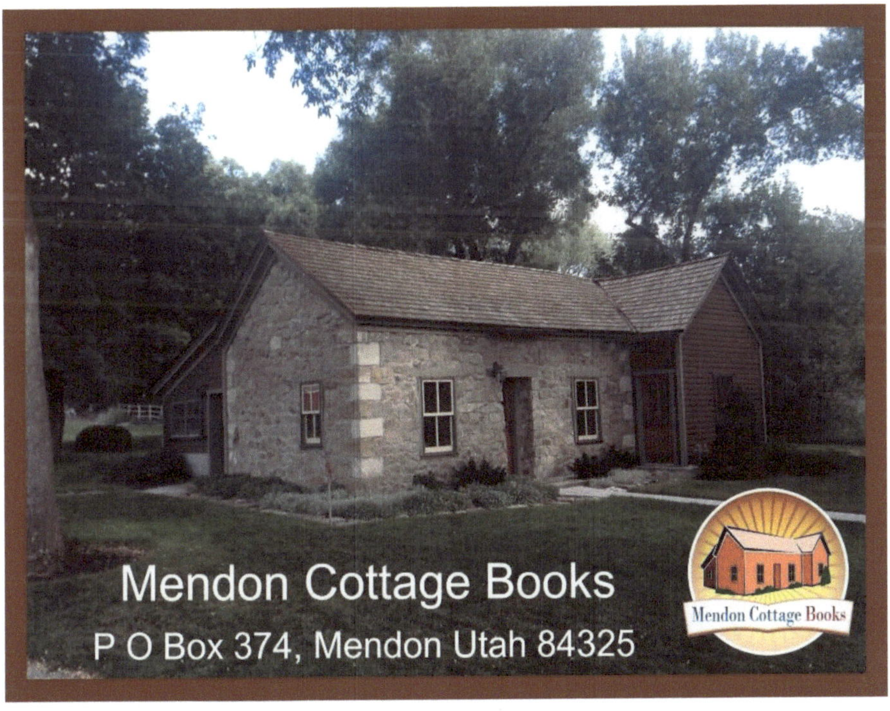

Mendon Cottage Books
P O Box 374, Mendon Utah 84325
Mendon Cottage Books

www.ingramcontent.com/pod-product-compliance
Lightning Source LLC
Chambersburg PA
CBHW050848290526
45792CB00002B/567